Our Lives with Rheumatoid Arthritis

Our Lives with Rheumatoid Arthritis:
A Mother and Daughter Team

Dedication

To my daughter
Who is strong and beautiful beyond measure.

To my husband who has seen us through the good
times and the bad.
And who has made the bad so much better.

To all the men and women in the medical
profession who work so hard to eradicate
Rheumatoid Arthritis.

To all of our family and friends who have seen us to
the other side.

Introduction

This is our attempt to bring the reader into our lives, past and present, as we have experienced Rheumatoid Arthritis.

Rheumatoid arthritis, or as it is also known as, 'RA', has been an all pervasive illness in our lives.

It has filled my daughter and I collectively with severe physical pain and mental anguish.

At times, it has been a lonely illness. Lying in bed while life goes by; lying down not in peace, but in bone crushing physical pain.

At times, it has been an isolating illness because no one else in our circle of friends really knew what we were feeling because they didn't suffer from the disease.

My hope is that we can bring comfort, insight, and a sense of direction to the person who has just been told, "*You have rheumatoid arthritis*".

Contents

Chapter 1

My Daughter's Life with Rheumatoid Arthritis

Onset of RA

My daughter was 17 years old when she first displayed signs of RA. She was a junior in high school when it crept up on her.

I'll never forget dropping her off at the curb in front of her high school and telling her to get out. We were having a fight.

She opened the door and swung her legs outside of the car. She stumbled. Her legs gave out from under her.

I thought she was kidding, but then I saw her face and knew it was no joke. She regrouped, said she was ok and went off to class.

Getting Medical Help

This physical collapse happened a couple more times until I was convinced that she needed to see the doctor.

We went to our general practitioner. She ran some tests.

"You have very high inflammation scores. I think you have Rheumatoid Arthritis," the doctor deduced. We were referred to a rheumatologist for follow-up.

We couldn't get into the rheumatologist for 8 weeks. My daughter's pain by this time was pervasive and unrelenting.

She experienced joint burn and what she described as a crucifixion-like tearing of her limbs.

I tried everything imaginable to try to bring relief to my daughter's agony.

I applied arthritis patches, creams, and lotions to her joints, limbs, feet and back.

I read every natural book on the subject. And then I attacked the health food store.

I got fish oils (but, she experienced nausea). I tried sulphur compounds that were specifically formulated for RA (she found out she was allergic to sulphur). I gave her vitamins and minerals specifically for RA (she broke out in hives).

She saw a holistic doctor and was given many garlic colonics.

She saw an acupuncturist and was poked and prodded with needles. He also used a sucking machine on her joints that made her scream. It left her skin purple at the joints.

Dealing with an out of control disease made her feel helpless. But one thing she could control was her diet.

She chose to become a vegetarian at this time after reading that a lot of illnesses could be eradicated with a change in diet. She is still on this diet.

We finally got in to see the rheumatologist. She confirmed my daughter had RA. I put my head down and held back the tears.

During that 8 week waiting period I was reading everything I could get my hands on regarding rheumatoid arthritis.

What stuck out in my mind when I heard the confirmation was 'shortened lifespan' and 'deformities'.

On the drive home my daughter asked me what was wrong. I told her what I knew. She groaned, "Oh no", and started to cry.

We both cried. Then I rallied and said, "Something will come along to help you." And at that moment I really felt that was true.

I was always my daughter's biggest cheerleader and I wasn't about to let this illness deprive her of a future.

I was determined, along with a mother's love, that she was going to make it to her wedding and give her dad and I grandchildren.

Her Journey

Her journey was just beginning as we made our way to UCLA for the Prosorba Column. This device cleanses the blood much like Dialysis cleans the kidneys.

My daughter went to this treatment every Friday for 3 months.

While on the Prosorba Column she developed an allergy to Benadryl. This was key because the procedure couldn't be done without it.

The treatment proved unsuccessful for my daughter even though the Prosorba team was working around the Benadryl allergy. They gave it their best shot.

Amid extreme pain and suffering, my daughter valiantly went from doctor to doctor seeking relief.

She was on Methotrexate and Plaquenil which afforded little relief. She added Enbrel and felt depressed so she switched to Humira. With Humira she had minimal relief.

It wasn't until she was prescribed Orencia that, mercifully, her pain stopped.

It has been a long haul, but she's finally been pain free for a year. She is 32. She had been suffering for 14 years before Orencia.

During those 14 years, she was homeschooled during the remainder of her junior year and her entire senior year. Through sheer determination she went on to Junior College.

On and off the pain became unbearable, so she spent many days alone in her room.

With the help of Orencia she now has plans to be a cosmetologist.

Luckily, she didn't suffer the deformities to her hands that are so characteristic of RA. Well, that's not completely true.

She had some damage that required surgery, but it wasn't Ulnar Drift. It was the dropping of her pinkies. She has scars, but her hands are fully mobile.

Orencia has slowed any potential damage that was on the way.   Her pinkies were starting to droop before the Orencia.

Family Support

My daughter always had a lot of help from the family.

My husband's aunt lived with us and she would tirelessly wait on my daughter. She would rub her feet for hours to rid her of some of her pain.

Her grandmother would make her favorite vegetarian dishes.

Well meaning family members were always on call to lend a sympathetic ear.

My husband and I made sure she got the care she needed.

Peer Support

My daughter was a popular girl all throughout grammar school and middle school. But, her junior year proved a challenge.

Many of her girlfriends didn't know the first thing about Rheumatoid Arthritis. Some actually thought she was faking it to try to get out of daily attendance at school.

Ignorance on their part proved very hurtful for my daughter.

The one saving grace was a boy she started seeing as a sophomore. He professed his love for her and stuck by her through her journey.

The Seasons of our life

Everyone has many seasons to their lives. My daughter's seasons were affected at a young age by Rheumatoid Arthritis.

From junior high school, through senior high school, through young adulthood, my daughter had these milestones affected by RA.

During the time span which would have included dating, college, and possible marriage, my daughter didn't participate in the normal progression of events.

With the exception of her boyfriend, she was always unfairly left out because of her Rheumatoid Arthritis.

Fortunately, Orencia proved to be the saving grace. Now my daughter is earnestly trying to play catch up with her life.

She can't go back and recapture her young adulthood with all of its aspects, but she can move forward and take advantage of every pain free moment.

The Outcome

Whatever her life path, I know that she has learned valuable lessons from her experience with Rheumatoid Arthritis.

She is stronger, more compassionate, and more aware of living in the moment than she would have been without this very painful experience.

Chapter 2

My Life with Rheumatoid Arthritis

Onset of RA

Rheumatoid Arthritis came on suddenly in my late 40's. I woke up one day and my legs were red and swollen. I couldn't walk. It was difficult to move.

My joints were on fire. I felt I was being torn apart at the joints when I would try to move.

When my family realized I was acting just like my daughter had acted, my family drove me to the hospital.

I went to emergency. I was seen and admitted into the hospital. While in the hospital, the doctor ran the usual tests.

He came to me after the second day and said that he was sending me to a rheumatologist.

My heart sank. My daughter still wasn't out of the woods with *her* RA. Orencia wasn't available yet.

Getting Medical Help

I was discharged with pain medication and I made the appointment with the rheumatologist.

He started me on Methotrexate. I ended up back in the hospital. Like my daughter, I was allergic to it. And like my daughter I'm allergic to sulphur. I also tried Humira and Enbrel self injectables - no luck.

My Journey

Unfortunately, during the time I was coming up empty with medications, the RA was whipping through my body like a firestorm.

As a result, I have the Ulnar Drift. That's when your fingers and toes turn either to the right or left away from their respective thumb or big toe.

16

I remember I took my daughter on a driving trip to Balboa Island. There was a quaint ice cream store we spotted and I stepped in.   An older woman waited on me,

I noticed her hands. I recognized them from a book I read on Rheumatoid Arthritis. She had complete Ulnar Drift. Her hands looked like seal fins.

My heart sank when I thought this is what my daughter will have to face one day.

Little did I know it was I who would be facing this obstacle.

In spite of three surgeries, I have deformed hands and feet. Thank goodness I'm right handed because my right hand is my better hand.

I can't pick things up with my hands like I used to. Also, my feet have gone from a shapely size 10 to an ugly size 11 wide.   My husband used to call my feet doll feet.

Family Support

I can't tell you how important family support was and is in my illness. Their sympathetic ears are very comforting.

I have physical help from my husband's family in the form of coming in to my house twice a month to clean the house. Also, my husband's aunt does the laundry.

In addition to the love and support of family members, what I desperately needed was the right medicine.

My husband played a pivotal role in my treatment. He always made sure the health insurance was paid.

This insurance allowed my daughter and I to start the Orencia infusion.

We have excellent insurance, but our premium was and is very high. We have our own business and our corporate rate is $2,600 a month.

Don't let that dissuade you from getting help. There are a lot of insurance companies that are affordable and they do cover rheumatoid infusions and drugs.

Orencia to the Rescue

For the past year I have been on Orencia. It is proving to be very effective for me. No pain.

All my lab reports show that my body is functioning optimally with the exception of my liver.

I had a liver biopsy because my tests warranted it. The liver biopsy came back normal.

I have a fatty liver which means I need exercise and a change in diet; two items that are within my control.

The Outcome

Today I experience happiness that transcends my illness.

I know where I could be pain wise, where I am, and I feel gratitude that I have found a mode of treatment that has freed me to have a life.

Unlike my daughter, I was able to go through more seasons of my life before Rheumatoid Arthritis hit me.

I had my high school years and college. I married, had my daughter, took care of my elderly mother, and travelled before RA took its toll on me. For this I am very grateful.

The Mother and Daughter Team

We are the ultimate mother and daughter team - bound by a painful life experience.

What we share now is a special bond.

We have the love, the closeness, the camaraderie that only happens between two people who've been through a long, arduous journey that creates that special bond.

A bond born out of pain.

A bond that is everlasting.

<u>Conclusion</u>

You are never really healed from Rheumatoid Arthritis. But, there is a great infusion drug that we use to keep our pain at bay.

My daughter and I are both grateful for Orencia and all the benefits we have been afforded because of this infusion.

We are both riding the cusp of these revolutionary new medications. We are anxious to see what is coming down the pipeline.

We are always thankful to have been born in the time we have been born into.

We shudder at the thought of being born in an earlier era.

We know very well that our lives would be horribly, radically different.

Resources

Arthritis Foundation

http://www.arthritis.org/rheumatoid-arthritis.php

Rheumatoid Arthritis

http://en.wikipedia.org/wiki/Rheumatoid_arthritis

Orencia

http://www.orencia.com/index.aspx

Notes

Notes

Notes